How to Successfully Implement Clinical Pathways

A step by step guide

Amanda Layton
Graham Morgan
Gary McHardy
Liz Allison

Kingsham

First published in 2002
by Kingsham Press

Oldbury Complex
Marsh Lane
Easthampnett
Chichester, West Sussex
PO18 OJW
United Kingdom

Typeset in AGaramond

Printed and bound by
MPG Books
Bodmin
Cornwall
United Kingdom

ISBN: 1-904235-07-7

British Library Cataloging in Publication Data
A catalogue record of this book is available from the British Library

About the authors

Amanda Layton is Head of the London Learning Partnership. Amanda trained as a nurse and has worked in quality improvement since 1989. She led on Pathway development at Central Middlesex Hospital as part of the Patient Focused project team during the early 1990s. In 1999 she moved to lead Phase 1 of the Cancer Services Collaborative in West London and is now working for London Region in the Modernisation Unit as a trainer and facilitator in quality improvement.

Graham Morgan is Director of Nursing and Quality at North West London Hospitals NHS Trust (NWLHT). In January 1995 Graham was appointed to the post of Executive Director of Nursing and Quality for North West London Hospitals NHS Trust. He is a frequent speaker at national and international conferences, and has conducted workshops in Finland and Sweden under the auspices of the Congress of the European Association of Hospital Managers. He is the author of a number of journal articles and is a contributor to two books on multi-disciplinary managed care. His particular interest is in multi-disciplinary team building and enhanced roles across professional boundaries. He was created a Knight Bachelor by Her Majesty The Queen in the Year 2000 Birthday's Honours List for services to health care.

Gary McHardy is Clinical Governance Facilitator at North West London Hospitals NHS Trust (NWLHT). Gary trained as an RGN and worked as a staff nurse on a variety of acute wards whilst also taking the lead in developing and implementing clinical pathways as the nurse representative. He joined the Quality team in 1999 where he further led the development of clinical pathways with a particular emphasis on the primary/secondary care interface. He recently co-led a lung cancer service redesign project for the nationally funded collaborative which was cited in the Cancer Plan.

Liz Allison is Clinical Redesigner BECAD at North West London Hospitals NHS Trust (NWLHT). Liz trained as a RGN at St. Thomas's Hospital. After qualifying in 1992, she moved to Central Middlesex Hospital where in 1994 she helped set up the Acute Assessment Unit and in 1997 the Critical Care Unit where much of the care was managed using clinical pathways and extended skills. Liz joined the Quality team in 1998, where the emphasis is to focus on redesign and to manage process using pathways as a key tool. She also worked with the London Learning Partnership, part of the NHS Learning Network, to create and support a group of clinicians interested in improving acute services by spreading good practice across the London region. She is currently leading on the clinical redesign of the new acute hospital at Central Middlesex.

Contents

Introduction ix

Getting started

Acknowledge and understand the reasons for change 3
Top down commitment and bottom ownership 4
Leadership of the project 5
The role of a facilitator 5
Project management 6
Design of the pathway 6
Choosing the case types and scope 8

Developing the pathway

Preparation 9
Collate background information 10
Who do you involve? 10
How do you get them written? 11
Agreeing milestones 14
Who approves the finished pathway? 14
Helpful hints 15
Difficulties to be aware of 15
Resources required 16

Implementation – getting it working

Training – pre-implementation 17
Content of training session – start from basics 17
Implementation issues 18
Helpful hints: 19
Difficulties to be aware of: 20
Resources required: 20

Evaluation – variance analysis

A technical term 20
Role of the case manager 22
Data analysis example 22
Helpful hints 24
Difficulties to be aware of 24
Resources required 24

The benefits of clinical pathway implementation

Predictable, high-quality care 25
Resource implications 26
Human resource implications 28

Further reading 30

Appendices

Appendix A: Asthma Protocol (Integrated Care Pathway) . . . 31
Appendix B: Collaborative Care IV Protocol 45
(Hospital at Home Integrated Care Pathway)

Introduction

This workbook aims to take you step by step through the process of developing and implementing your first pathway. It is based on considerable experience over the last 10 years of introducing them at Central Middlesex Hospital, now known as The North West London Hospitals NHS Trust.

Section 1

GETTING STARTED

Acknowledge and understand the reasons for change

The Labour government of 1997 in a white paper for the NHS introduced the statutory duty for quality improvement at local level – Clinical Governance. Patients, and Trust Boards are ever more mindful of the need for a service which is able to produce predictable quality care. Yet how many providers of health care can produce a document which sets out clearly what the plan of care for a given condition will be? How many thousands of hip replacements are performed each year, and yet health care organisations are unable to provide patients with a plan of intended interventions. Do we really believe that the most efficient way of working is to make it up anew each time a patient arrives at our door? We continue to structure our work as if every case were the exception rather than the rule.

The majority of what we do is routine. What we did yesterday, we do today and will do tomorrow. By reinventing the process each time we work inefficiently, we occasionally omit various parts of high quality evidence based care, and duplicate others, lowering the quality of the outcome. The planning and documenting of care in the traditional way is inefficient, and needlessly repetitious. How often does a doctor do a round and document the plan of care in the 'medical case records'. The nurse, and if required the therapist then updates their plan and documents what the doctor has said on the round. How often does a profession gain access to, or read another professionals record? If we are to deliver predictable quality care, then we have to maximise the use of inevitably limited resources. Approaching the planning and recording of care in a multi-disciplinary manner will assist in achieving the goal, which is surely the desire of all of us in the health service, to simplify the process, reduce variation, and achieve good quality outcomes at the lowest possible cost.

These desires are described in the First Class Service (DOH 1998) – delivering consistent high quality care. It is about process and systems. It is often the way systems are designed that determines the outcomes, individuals rarely fail. The aim is to anticipate events by planning and managing process in a proactive way. Lots of experience with clinical pathways has confirmed what most people involved in the delivery of healthcare already know – that is a high percentage of clinical activity is predictable. Mapping out the process across the multi-professional groups is a surer way of managing and monitoring activity and consequently managing risk.

Top down commitment and bottom ownership

The Chief Executive, senior clinical staff and members of the Board, should share with staff at the 'sharp end' a vision of the changes they seek to bring about, set within the framework of the overall strategy of the organisation. They need to know what is going on, show a clear commitment to the introduction of the clinical pathways, and be prepared to provide the resources necessary to bring about the change. Resources such as a facilitator, secretarial time, printing and photocopying facilities and most importantly time for staff to develop the clinical pathways.

Even if there is top down commitment, change will never really stick if the people who are to implement it see it only as something being imposed from above. They must first come to an understanding and acknowledge the need for change, and then be responsible for driving it forward. Staff are past masters at not following systems imposed by above. Never forget that implementing a pathway is fundamentally about CHANGE.

Among the changes involved in this new way of planning and documenting care are:

- the way staff consider their work
- the way staff record their work
- the way staff communicate
- the information the patient and their relatives can access

The following points are seen as critical elements in the process:

- openness and honesty with staff
- an opportunity for staff to discuss their concerns
- a view about 'where it is heading'
- an emphasis with staff that it is 'theirs to own'

The importance of *listening* to staff cannot be over emphasised. Staff are somewhat cynical about 'new initiatives' and success must be seen as a priority not only for the project but to give something back to the participating staff.

Leadership of the project

Who the leader will be is dependent on the culture pertaining within the organisation. Some sites will choose to have a dedicated steering committee, others could adopt different structures using ones already in place such as the quality or audit committee. What should not be forgotten is that **this is a clinical initiative and must be clinically led**.

More recently individuals have been identified to lead and co-ordinate such a project eg pathway facilitators.

The role of a facilitator

This person needs to be FACILITATOR, CO-ORDINATOR and EVANGELIST for the project. Good people skills are essential as are organisational abilities. For the project to have credibility within the organisation it is important that the role is seen as being a senior one within the organisation. Their skills need to include:

- clinical credibility
- good communication skills
- professionally 'neutral'
- patience
- enthusiasm
- breadth of vision
- assertiveness

The responsibilities of the facilitator include:

- spreading the word about pathways throughout the organisation
- motivating the staff involved and listening to their concerns
- facilitating pathway writing and variance analysis sessions
- challenging long held assumptions about what care is given, by whom, when and where
- training of staff for the pilot
- ensuring that the pathway recording and variance tracking is being performed correctly
- working alongside or liaising with audit staff about the variance analysis data.
- teaching and encouraging Directorate staff to become self-sufficient.

- liaison with Senior Management about the strategic direction of the project.
- attendance at any Hospital Steering Group meetings
- liaison with all staff members involved with the pilot
- ensuring supply of pathways in required areas
- once several pathways are in use, ensure they are regularly reviewed and that the most recent version is being used.

Project management

It is essential to have sound project management and important to keep up the momentum.

As with any project, clear plans and time goals both focus the mind and help keep one heading in the right direction with timed goals.

Stages along the project plan will include:

- developing a team with shared aims
- agreed case types
- scope of boundary for the pathway
- pathway design and writing phases
- implementation dates for each case type
- training dates for implementation and variance analysis training
- variance feed back and review of pathway.

Design of the pathway

It is best to agree the overall design or framework of the clinical pathway at a local unit level, as ownership is key to a successful change process. Pathways developed at another site should only be used to stimulate debate and discussion. Even if at the end of this discussion it is decided to use the document substantially unchanged, the process staff go through in agreeing on a final version is critical to successful implementation.

When designing the framework it is helpful to bear these points in mind:

- **Reappraise current models of documentation.**
  What then should happen to other means of documentation which are currently in use? Should every thing be removed to

make way for the new system, or should the two run in tandem for a short period of time? Any decision as to what approach should be adopted can only be taken with due regard to circumstances applying to individual sites. If implemented as a duplicate system, on top of existing models of care, time spent in documentation increases. Some sites may choose to do this as an interim, however it is harder to get staff to use the pathways if they are also documenting in their 'own' notes.

- **Design to be the 'actual' document of care**
  Pathways designed to be the 'actual' document of care do lead to a reduction in documentation time. The act of creating the pathway as the record of care, also reinforces the need for staff to refer to the document.

- **Identify process interventions and outcomes within a time frame.**
  The pathways need to make explicit the clear link between what is done, and when. Time frames may be minutes, hours, days, weeks, or when an outcome has been met.

- **Exception reporting.**
  Designed to encourage reporting by exception makes any detour from the pathway that much easier to identify. It also reduces documentation time.

- **Design a user friendly framework.**
  They should be clear, precise and not overcrowded with information. Cross referencing to organisation wide core care quality standards is adopted by some Trusts as a method of providing backup information without overcrowding the document.

- **Design to include clearly identifiable milestones – key outcomes of care**
  These are key steps in the process of care and are also used as the basis for collecting concurrent audit data.

Example of pathway design

Patient name | **DAY 1** | Hospital no

MILESTONES/OUTCOMES	MET	If no please give reason and action
• Oral or IV steroids given < 1 hour	❑	
• Inhaled steroids commenced	❑	
• SaO_2 >95% on O_2	❑	
• PEFR recorded at least 4 hourly	❑	

ASSESSMENT		Yes	No
• Unable to speak sentences		❑	❑
• Central cyanosis		❑	❑
• Arterial saturation < 95% on O_2		❑	❑
• Tachycardia > 110/mins		❑	❑
• Respiratory rate > 25/min		❑	❑
• Evidence of CO_2 retention	**If Yes refer to ITU Registrar**	❑	❑
• Poor level of consciousness	**If Yes refer to ITU Registrar**	❑	❑

• Observations: TPR and BP 6 hourly (if stable)
Peak Flow pre and post nebuliser
Pulse Oximetry (O_2 concentration _____ %)

Urinalysis for glucose on admission ________________________________

INVESTIGATIONS	Yes	No	Comments		
• Chest X-ray	❑	❑	Pneumothorax	Consolidation	Normal
• Sputum for culture	❑	❑	Hyperexpanded		
• FBC	❑	❑			
• U&Es	❑	❑			
• Repeat ABGs **IF**	❑	❑	Ph	PCO_2	PO_2
Initially abnormal or O_2 sats on air < 92%			HCO_3		
• Theophylline levels if relevant:	❑	❑			

DRUGS	Yes	No
• Commence inhaled steroids	❑	❑

OTHER MANAGEMENT		Yes	No
• **Oxygen therapy** (in high concentrations as necessary consider humidification)	_______ %	❑	❑
• **Refer to physio**		❑	❑
• **Care plan** discussed and explained to patient by:	______________________ (sign)		

ADDITIONAL INFORMATION

RGN: AM | PM | Night

Choosing the case types and scope

In deciding which case types should be chosen for a successful pilot the following needs to be kept in mind:

- confine pathway to one case or area
- the level of predictability
- enthusiastic staff – especially medical and nursing staff.

Staff working on the unit have their own ideas as to which case types they wish to work on, and it is best to allow them to make the choice. Once a Trust-wide roll-out is planned then the criteria is usually for case types which are:

- high volume
- high cost
- high risk
- large volume of evidence based research.

Most case types are suitable to be managed using a pathway, but there needs to be a clear strategy on how senior personnel within the organisation wish to roll-out in a Trust-wide initiative. The guidance should come from the Trust Board or Clinical Governance Steering Committee.

Determining the scope of the pathway by having a clear start and end point, ensures all staff are working towards the same goal. Pathways are not just for inpatient management. They are also used in a variety of settings. For example:

- from GP to outpatients – to improve referral process from primary care
- for the management of chronic conditions across the health economy
- from GP to the operating theatre and discharge for planned surgery.

The complexity of developing a pathway that encompasses the whole patient journey and as such crosses many health care agencies can be underestimated. For this reason you may choose to take a staged approach with the scope of the pathway i.e. referral, treatment & discharge stages. A seamless service can then be achieved by linking these processes.

DEVELOPING THE PATHWAY

Preparation

You have chosen your case type and have ensured that you have top down commitment. You are ready to start developing your first pathway.

It is necessary to do some background preparation before starting:

- Collate background information
- Consider who to involve in the project

Collate background information

A literature search for evidence, research, consensus statements, or nationally agreed guidelines should be carried out, so that current best practice can be incorporated in the pathways. Examples include Royal College of Physicians guidelines for the management of Fractured Neck of Femur, and the British Thoracic Societies Guidelines for the management of acute asthma. Organisational priorities should also be considered.

A baseline audit should be carried out in order that any improvements that are made by the introduction of a pathway are able to be clearly shown.

Who do you involve?

Essentially the staff who deliver care. Examples include: pharmacists; nurses; doctors; therapists; radiographers; radiologists; primary care staff and anaesthetists. These may be junior or senior members of the team. There are benefits to both.

What is important is that whilst everyone cannot be involved in the actual writing of the pathway, *all* staff should have the opportunity to participate at some level. A way of achieving maximum ownership within a unit is to have a 'larger' group meeting less frequently to agree which case-types and to approve the pathway, and a smaller group who meet to write the pathway.

The choice of staff who are involved in writing the pathway should represent the case type chosen. From a practical point of view between 4 to 8 individuals is recommended, in order to achieve discussion and consensus.

Involving patient views is also advised. This may be in the form of patient surveys, focus groups or having a user on the pathway working group.

How do you get them written?

Mapping out the *current* process

There is not one way for writing them, although representatives of the team should meet on at least one occasion to discuss and approve the pathway. Included below are different methods that could be used:

Method 1

Prior to the first pathway meeting for an agreed case-type, each team member is provided with a blank pathway, and asked to fill in their own contribution to the care process. These are then collated by the facilitator, and a draft copy of the pathway is made and distributed at the meeting for discussion, comment and a consensus is to be achieved.

Method 2

The facilitator and team members meet and use the agreed pathway framework on a flip chart or board, to draft out the anticipated outcomes and process of care for the chosen case type. This is then typed up and distributed for comments.

Method 3

The facilitator and team members meet and using a flip chart and post it notes they flow chart the process of care and identify the anticipated outcomes for the given case type. This is then drawn together by the facilitator within an agreed framework. This has an advantage as post-it notes can be moved if additions to the process are identified.

Method 4

Case notes for a given case type are retrospectively audited to identify the process of care delivered to patients who have already undergone treatment. The processes are then drawn up within the agreed framework, and discussed and debated by the team.

Comments:

There are advantages and disadvantages to each method. A great deal of time can be spent finding the right words/phrases to put in the agreed framework, particularly for more complex case-types, leading to potential difficulties with methods 1 & 2 as time is taken up by the staff because of this. The less structured method 3 can allow more time for debate of the more fundamental issues of process and outcome, but requires a greater amount of the facilitators time to apply the flow chart text to a framework. Method 4 provides valuable baseline data, but is the most time consuming.

Redesigning the process of care

It should be remembered that pathways should be seen as a tool for change and not just documenting care in a new way. It is the role of the facilitator to gently challenge assumptions and current ways of working to help identify areas for redesign and improvement. Often duplication of staff roles and other inefficiencies in the system become apparent during this phase of the process. Key questions the facilitator can use which will help draw this out include:

- What is the most appropriate care?
- When is the most appropriate time?
- Who is the most appropriate person?
- Where is the most appropriate place?

What is the most appropriate care?

This question is fundamentally about what is the evidence base for our clinical decision making. It is about assessing the strength of research and the putting the findings into practice.

Of course there are many areas of clinical and organisational practice that have little evidence to support practice or the evidence base is conflicting. This is an opportunity for the experts within the pathway group to describe the standard of care they would wish to meet.

But, obtaining a consensus can be one of the most challenging aspects of pathway design. Individual clinicians have differing views on certain aspects of care. Where there is no evidence it is best to arrive at a consensus of recognised best practice, if necessary benchmarking against other organisations. Ultimately it will be the responsibility of the clinical lead to ensure that the pathway reflects a standard of care that will reduce the variation for the patient. Special dispensation for individual clinicians should be avoided.

When is the most appropriate time?

Traditionally many aspects of patient care is arranged around the organisation itself. For example, why are so many wound drains removed on a Monday morning on surgical wards? Because that is when the ward round happens. In an ideal world the drain removal or any other procedure would be carried out when the patient is ready. That is, when the patient has met the agreed outcome.

So when challenging the current pathway of care we are trying to identify what is the patient outcome needed to progress the patient on to the next stage of care e.g. drainage < 30 mls in 24 hours.

Who is the most appropriate person?

This question is about who has the skills to carry out an aspect of care safely. If we take the example above, the criteria that a surgeon would use for removal of a drain may be <30 mls drainage in 24 hours. The decision-making skill is about applying this criteria. A nurse has the skills and knowledge to assess 24 hour drainage, as the nurse is closest to the patient at the appropriate time, the nurse should be empowered to make the decision to remove the drain. Training needs of staff may also be identified

Where is the most appropriate place?

A major benefit arising from the national interest in redesigning clinical care is that it has allowed us to ask the question, where could this element of care be delivered?

Thus the focus for rehabilitation has moved from an acute hospital setting to the patients home. Likewise patients with drains or catheters in situ can be appropriately managed at home. This shift to shorten length of hospital stay will push the boundaries even further whilst maintaining safety.

Agreeing milestones

Once the new process of care has been designed, milestones (key outcomes of care) should be agreed. They are key steps in the patient pathway which need to be met before the patient can move safely onto the next stage of the pathway. It is these agreed milestones that are then used as the audit tool.

Milestones should be:

- Evidence based
- Critical steps in the process
- Areas of great variation
- Priorities for the organisation

Example of milestones from Stroke Pathway

Day One

Milestones:	Met	If not met give reasons:
CT scan ordered	☐	
Swallow assessment commenced	☐	
Anti-embolism stockings in place	☐	

Day Two

Milestones:	Met	If not met give reasons:
Plan for hydration initiated	☐	
Aspirin commenced	☐	

Who approves the finished pathway?

Prior to implementation, the pathways require approval and agreement by the senior members of the team, the consultant, charge nurse and other relevant professionals.

How long does this process take?

The first pathway will invariably take more time than subsequent ones, due to the learning curve of all concerned and for some the agreement of a framework. Time will also vary with the complexity of the case-type.

A fairly predictable and straightforward case type can take approximately 3 to 4 hours to prepare a first draft. Examples of these include: Grommets, Transurethral Resection of the Prostate and Total Hip Replacement.

Pathway example

See Appendices A and B.

Helpful hints

- Start with something simple and relatively straightforward, it is important that it is a success.
- Keep the momentum up, don't take too long over this process, people need to see the results of their work.
- Date and code the pathway, so that when it is updated at a later date there is a record of each version. This is important for legal reasons.
- Develop pathways for patients and their families using less 'jargonised' language. These help provide information, and encourage patient participation. With some imagination they can be designed and used by children on the paediatric wards to colour in when an intervention or outcome has been met.

Difficulties to be aware of

- The limitation of time – particularly of those in the clinical area. It is helpful to keep meetings to time and to ensure they are productive. Some staff may need to be encouraged to keep quiet whilst others may need to be drawn out. These are all skills required of the facilitator.
- Resistance and reluctance to sharing information. Anxieties over roles and cross-training may lead some staff to being extremely vague about the activities that they undertake.
- Reluctant medical staff. Involve them when they believe they have something unique to contribute. Highlight areas which will be of particular interest to them, such as clinical audit data, the possible use of the pathway for research purposes, and improved documentation of patient care.

- Getting the case type right. If you are experiencing problems it may be that you have been too broad or not broad enough in the definition of the case-type.

Resources required

- **Access to a computer and typing skills.**
  This is to design the framework and type in the pathway. Word processing packages with tables such as Microsoft® Word are quite satisfactory.

- **Access to a meeting room and copious supplies of caffeine**

- **Staff time:**
  This will depend on the method adopted and the complexity of the case-type. At the outset of the project this part may take longer.

  To draft a relatively straight forward pathway:
  - Approximately three 1 hour meetings with 4–8 staff
  - 6–10 hours of facilitators/secretaries time for typing
  - time should also be accounted for communicating with team and organising meetings

IMPLEMENTATION – GETTING IT WORKING

The initial input and follow up support at this stage in the process is frequently underestimated. A common assumption particularly of senior staff is that once the pathways are written that is the end of it! This is not the case. Pathway development is not purely about the paper/electronic document – it is primarily about change and people.

People exhibit resistance to change in differing ways. The training and support that is necessary in the implementation stage needs to address professionals anxieties. This can be supported by ensuring that their voices are heard, and promoting ownership of the project.

Support and training needs to start before the implementation date, and continued following implementation with intense support.

Training – pre-implementation

- This is best carried out as close to implementation as possible.
- Arrange a number of sessions so that the majority of staff from the multidisciplinary team can attend (approximately 3 meetings of 30–45 minutes held in the clinical area).
- Training sessions led by a member of staff on the unit if possible. This isn't always feasible and frequently the facilitator will do this. What is important is that staff are aware that there is commitment from senior members on the unit for their implementation.
- Provide each member of the team with a copy of the pathway or access to one, to familiarise themselves with it.

Content of training session – start from basics

The why

- Reasons for change
- Top down commitment
- Benefits of pathways for the patient and staff

How to use them

- **Individualisation**
  Pathways are written for the vast majority of patients who will require no additional interventions. On occasions when a patient has specific requirement of care, these can be added to the pathway by recording variance and recording free text evaluation of care within the pathway. For example diabetes, this can be added to the pathway by the member of the team undertaking the assessment. It needs to be made clear when and how to make these additions.

- **Charting variance**
  Staff may require reassurance that some variance from the pathway is anticipated as it only reflects the care needed for the majority of patients. The agreed method of charting variation needs to be clarified.

- **Signatures, where to write and what to write**
  The requirement for training input increases if the pathway has been designed to become the record of care and to replace other documentation.

- **Use in shift handover**
  To identify the activities and interventions anticipated for that day and any variations to the plan. They provide a useful tool for handover, consistent, precise and concise.

- **Placing a patient on a pathway**
  Clarify the criteria for starting a patient on a pathway and who is responsible for this.

- **Removing a patient from a pathway.**
  Sometimes a patient's condition varies so far from the predicted plan that the pathway fails to reflect a true picture of the management required. Examples of this include a cardiac arrest, or pulmonary embolus. Staff need to be clear what to do in these cases, which is to remove the management of the patient from the pathway, document the reason and a write a new plan of care.

Implementation issues

Role of the case manager

In order to ensure all care as agreed and identified on the pathway is carried out as planned, or remedial action is taken to keep the patient as close to the pathway as possible, an individual (who is often a member of the nursing staff) takes responsibility on a shift or daily basis to co-ordinate the team. This reinforces accountability. The case manager also takes a lead role in the collection of variance data.

Where is the pathway to be located

This is an important point to agree with the team. As a multidisciplinary document it needs to be accessible to all members of staff. In some cases the pathways are located at the end of the patient's bed, thus facilitating and enhancing patient participation. There are many advantages in adopting this approach, however, issues of confidentiality and the patient's wishes need to be considered. In many clinical areas, the pathway is located in a ring binder alongside the hospital notes folder in the patients trolley, The hospital notes are used purely as reference, and the ring binder becomes the live complete record of care. This approach has proved very successful.

Resistance from other professionals can occur if it is held in the 'nurses notes' or the 'medical notes'. Shared ownership of the document needs to be reinforced.

Supporting the staff

The change process can be stressful for staff, therefore support is required from the facilitator and senior staff at key times e.g. ward rounds and handover. Support can help to alleviate anxiety and provide valuable feedback. Don't be afraid to congratulate and encourage.

Collecting information

Record staff comments and suggestions during the pilot, but do not make changes unless care described is unsafe.

Review of pathways once implemented

- Analyse the pathway variances fairly quickly after initial implementation (i.e. 10–30 patients) to ensure that there are no problems in the content of the pathway. Audit results may also help get staff on board.
- Formally review them at regular periods, for example 6 monthly to ensure that they reflect any changes in practice. They are a legal document, and for legal purposes, old copies that have been updated should be filed and kept for future reference. Ideally keep a central record of all active and old updated pathways.

Helpful hints:

- Develop a simple 'Guidelines for use' document. This will help by reinforcing what was covered in the training session.
- Identify opinion leaders/key players. These staff help reinforce the training given and facilitate implementation.

- Invest in some continuing support. Its often helpful to have someone (the facilitator or identified opinion leaders) spend about an hour a day on the unit for a week or two following initial implementation to help iron out lingering concerns, and identify and deal with any covert resistance. Units that have opinion leaders generally require less support in this stage from the facilitator.
- Photocopy a limited number initially because there will be changes to the document.
- Limit minor changes to the pathways, as there is a tendency to keep making small changes to the document especially at the beginning when refinement to the tool is occurring.
- Adopt a coding system on the pathway so that it is clear that the most 'up to date' one is in use.

Difficulties to be aware of:

- Change brings with it a rise in uncertainty, and some covert resistance.
- People often have to hear something more than once to grasp a new concept
- This often takes longer than you think!

Resources required:

- 3–4 training sessions per new unit. This is not an ongoing resource.
- Some limited ongoing support. Either from the facilitator or key workers on the unit. Approximately 1 hour per day for an initial 2 weeks.
- Paper and photocopying for pathways

EVALUATION – VARIANCE ANALYSIS

By definition, a variance is simply a detour from the process, activities or outcomes specified on the pathway. It is an inevitable part of any process and it can occur anywhere. Because pathways reflect the care for the majority, some patient variances are to be expected.

Experience has taught us that staff will not document detailed reasons for every variance that occurs. By the introduction of key milestones and the monitoring of variance against these on a daily basis, we can at least be sure that the most significant steps in the patient pathway have been met, or if not why not.

All staff are asked to document variance as they occur against the agreed milestones and to record the reasons for the variance which is crucial for audit purposes.

Example: Major gynaecology surgery pathway post op Day 1

Milestones:	Met	If not met give reasons:
Tolerating light diet	☐	Vomiting post op anyti emetic not given pre op
Drain removed	☑	
Urethral catheter removed	☑	
PCA discontinued 36 hours post op	☐	Pt still c/o of pain on movement

Ways in which variance can be used

In contrast to traditional audit methods, the charting and analysis of variance provides both a concurrent and retrospective focus on the evaluation of care.

Concurrent variance

- enables the pathway to be dynamic not static
- provides a method for individualisation
- alerts the professional to the need to take action
- identifies the critical points where decisions are required
- is important from a legal point of view to identify why the agreed pathway has not been followed.

The concurrent charting of variance embeds staff in the audit cycle. It is not something that is just overlaid but is *integral* to the whole process and delivery of care, and adds a new 'here and now' dimension to audit. If a milestone has not been met due to clinician variance or a simple "omission", this can be corrected on the spot. If for example, an asthmatic patient is discharged home without steroids, the case manager can rectify the situation directly. This means that the patient does not miss out on vital evidence based healthcare.

Retrospective variance analysis

Following discharge, the variances are copied and aggregated for analysis by the multi-disciplinary team to:

- demonstrate an improved service
- identify opportunities for further improvement
- identify patterns and trends
- highlight areas where more focused audits are required
- highlight bottlenecks or weak points in a system
- demonstrate quality and cost impacts.

The most significant results are fed back to the department on a regular basis, and change if needed should be implemented. One benefit of this type of audit is that there is little time delay in the analysis of this data, and the staff involved in the analysis are the ones who have been delivering the care. This encourages ownership of the data, and staff are more likely to be actively involved in making any necessary changes. The focus of the data collection is to improve care, and this needs to be reinforced at all stages.

Role of the case manager

To ensure that the pathway is used and that key milestones of care are met and if not that they are correctly actioned. They can also be responsible for collecting the variance data on a concurrent basis.

Data analysis example

One way to analyse the data is to look at the number of patients who met the agreed milestones. And to ask of those that failed to meet the milestone, was it because of 'avoidable variance' or 'unavoidable variance'. It is the avoidable variances that the multi-disciplinary team need to focus their attention on in order to make any necessary changes to the system to improve patient care. It can also be helpful to show progress over time, demonstrating that the process of care is becoming more predictable (see Figures 1 and 2).

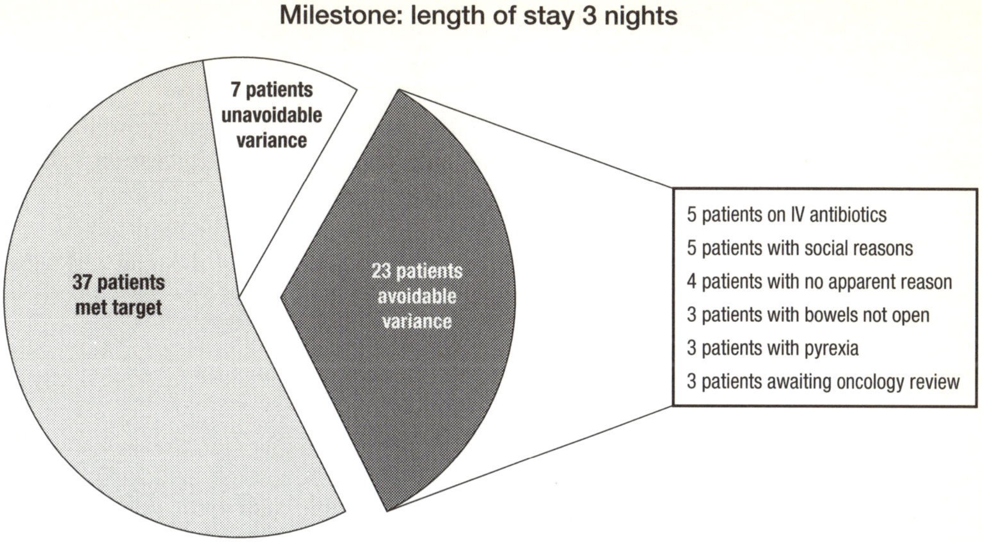

Figure 1 Major gynaecology pathway variance

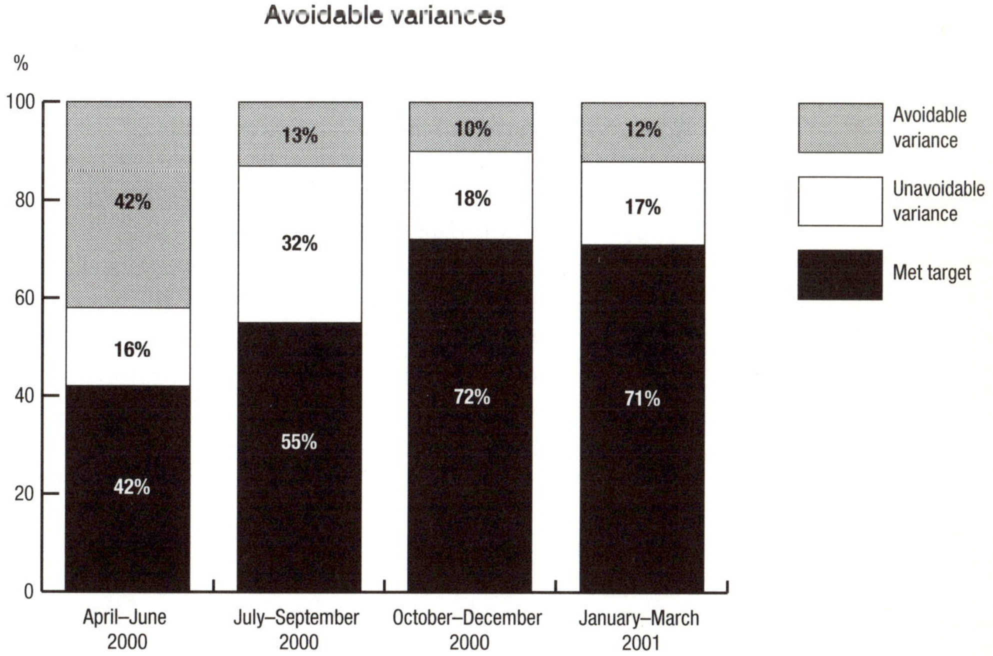

Figure 2 Major gynaecology: Central Middlesex Hospital

Helpful hints

- Analyse variances from a new pathway quickly.
- The process of analysing the variances with staff from the unit, provide another valuable opportunity for discussion, education and most importantly team building.
- Encourage staff from the unit to feedback the results to the rest of their team. This reinforces ownership of the data and helps any change process occur.
- Focus on patterns and trends.

Difficulties to be aware of

- Documenting variance. Frequently staff have difficulty with charting variance, both in how or where to document and in identifying the reasons why a variance occurred. It is helpful to focus training sessions on this area, and use examples. Following the first analysis of data, staff themselves often see the need for improved charting of variance as they start to want to know more and can be frustrated by the limited amount of documentation present.

Resources required

- **Access to a meeting room and of course caffeine!**

- **Staff time:**
  Initial training in variance analysis
  - 2–3 hour session, to train in the theory behind variance and to carry out variance analysis from the unit's first 10–20 cases.
  - Variance analysis – ongoing
  - Approximately one hour meeting of 3–6 staff to analyse their variances
  - 2–6 hours of facilitators/audit staff time for preparation of results
  - 1 hour feedback session for results to multidisciplinary team to agree action plan

- **Access to a computer**
  The data are initially best analysed by hand. However as more data are generated, some units find it helpful to use

spreadsheets or statistical packages for analysis. Results for presentation require use of a graphics and/or word processing package.

THE BENEFITS OF CLINICAL PATHWAY IMPLEMENTATION

Predictable, high-quality care

Natural forum for team building

The act of bringing staff together to discuss and evaluate their individual contributions in the delivery of care, provides a natural forum for increasing awareness and the opportunity to recognise the part each plays in the increasingly complex process of health care, whilst also highlighting overlap and repetition in work and the need of mutual dependence.

Part of such a process must be a conscious attempt at team building, with group working as the way to bring together the differing professional attitudes. If due regard is not taken in this area then changes may well occur in the first instance only to disappear shortly after. When changes occur we need to ensure that they stick.

Improved communication with patients

The majority of patients and their families like being more aware of what is going to happen to them, and feel a greater involvement in the process.

Improvements in quality of care and outcomes

Improvements in quality are achieved at all stages in the process, from meeting together to plan care, through to the audit of variance.

Clinical audit

The variance analysis data have led to a greater understanding and interest in the audit process.

Variances from pathways provide a practical mechanism for audit, they are collected concurrently, and as such are less time consuming. The audit process through charting variance becomes part of the routine practice of care. Aggregated they provide valuable multidisciplinary audit data. Variance trends can identify areas where more focused audit needs to be carried out, or where improvements in practice should be addressed.

Improved discharge planning

Pathways from admission focus staff, patients and their relatives attention on an anticipated date of discharge. Variances from the predicted process or outcomes of care highlight discharge problems at an early stage.

Resource implications

Reduction in length of stay

Significant reductions in overall length of stay for a number of case-types have been achieved (see Figure 3).

Reduction in documentation time

At Central Middlesex Hospital we demonstrated the reduction in time nurses spent documenting care through observational analysis. The results showed that following pathway implementation, there has been an overall reduction in documentation time from 14% to 6%, and a corresponding increase in time spent in direct patient care.

Improvements in predicting activity

Managing care using pathways allow one to predict far more accurately the day of discharge, as variability is reduced. This in turn helps in planning other organisational issues, for example operation bookings and managing bed occupancy (see Figures 4 and 5).

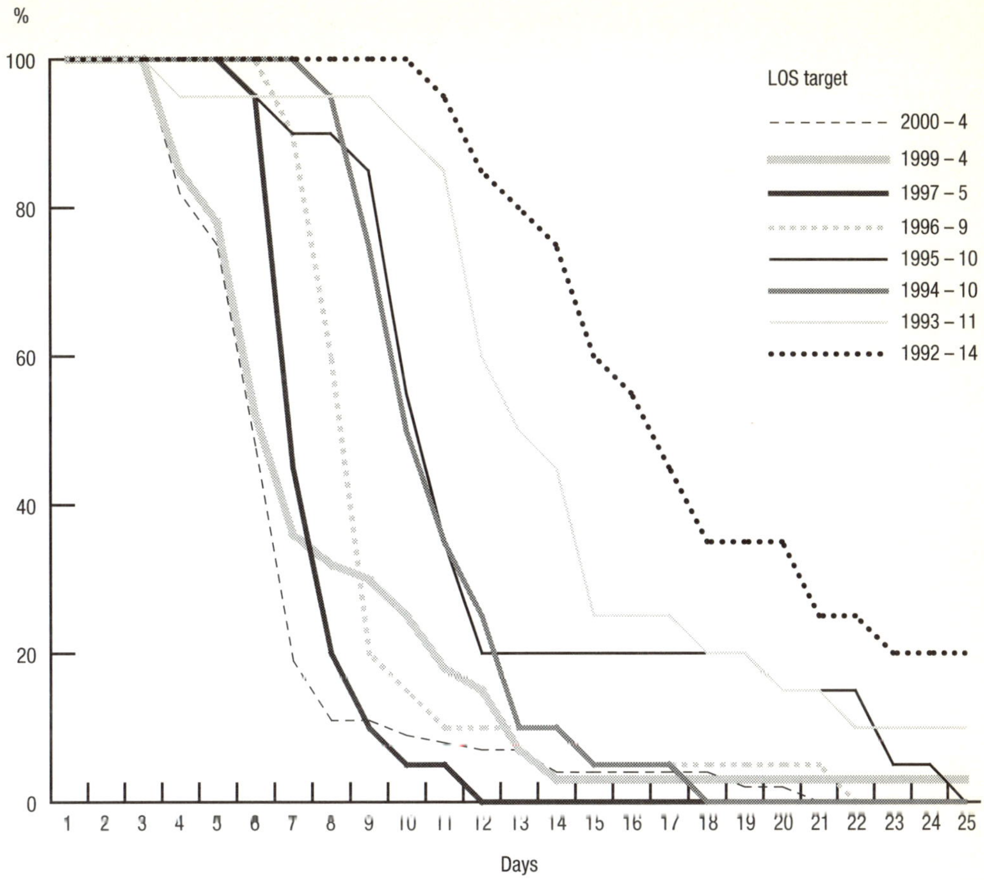

Figure 3 Bed occupancy – total hip replacement (%)

Knock on effects for other case-types

Changes in practice identified through developing one pathway or variance analysis often have positive quality, cost and time saving ramifications for other case types. Examples include: drug regimes, prophylaxis regimes, agreement of multi-skilling issues, and reductions in the admission process.

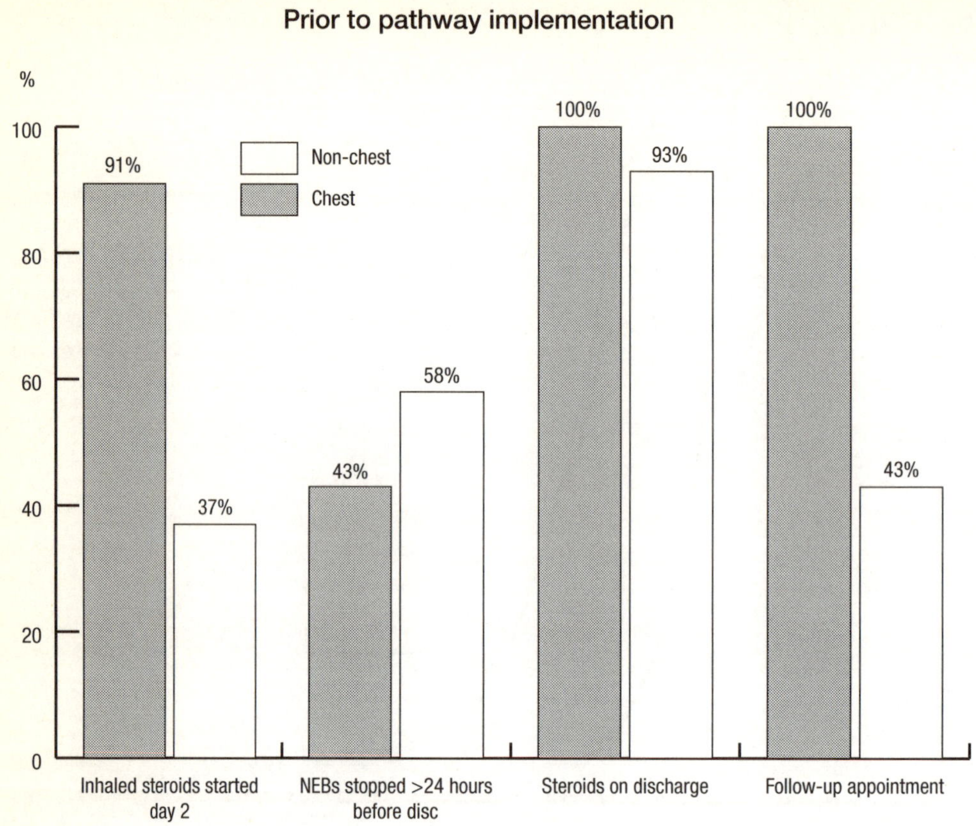

Figure 4 Variation in care

Human resource implications

A move to proactive care

Pathways provide the overall framework of care. Imparting this knowledge to ALL members of staff empowers them to become proactive in their management of care, instead of reactive. An example to illustrate this point, is bringing forward activities due to take place at a weekend, instead of delaying them.

Accountability reinforced

Registered staff have always been accountable for their actions. Managing care using an agreed pathway, reinforces accountability in a more clearly defined way. The use of clinical pathways is not

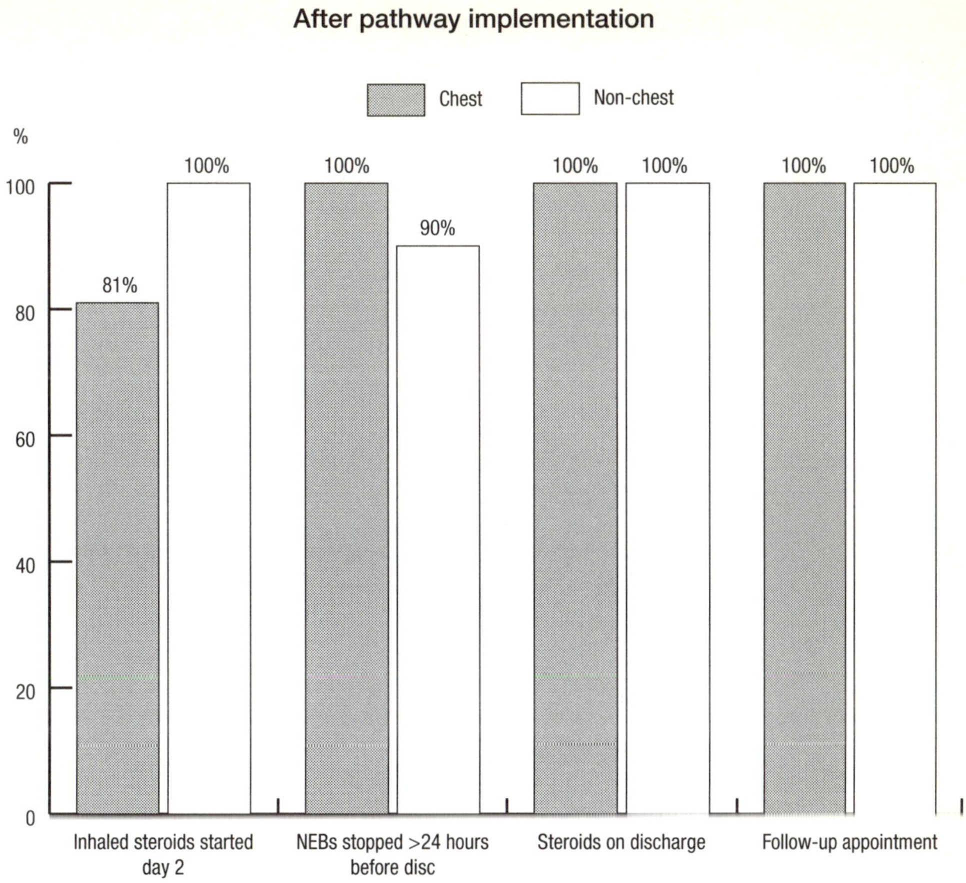

Figure 5 Variation in care

an excuse for leaving ones 'grey cells' elsewhere. If pathways are to be used intelligently for the benefit of patients then greater knowledge rather than less is required.

Identification of human resource issues

The process of care is made explicit with pathways, and as a consequence it is much easier to decipher (than using traditional plans of care where a great deal of detective work was required) whether the pathway has been followed, and/or appropriate action taken. It becomes easier to identify staff who have problems managing care, and to organise appropriate training programmes for them.

FURTHER READING

Developing Care Pathways – the handbook (book 1) & the tool kit (book 2) – Kathryn de Luc in collaboration with Denise Kitchiner, Amanda Layton, Elaine Morris, Yvonne Murray and Sue Overill. Oxford: Radcliffe Medical Press 2000.

The use of care pathways as tools to support the implementation of evidence-based practice – V.L. Currie & G. Harvey – *Journal of International Care,* Vol 14, No. 4, 2000

Integrated Care pathways: a Practical Approach to Implementation. Middleton S, Roberts A, eds. Oxford: Butterworth-Heinemann, 2000.

Layton A, Moss F, Morgan G. Mapping out the patient's journey: experiences of developing pathways of care. *QHC* 1998;7 (Supplement):S30–S36

APPENDICES

Appendix A: Asthma Protocol (Integrated Care Pathway)
Appendix B: Collaborative Care IV Protocol (Hospital at Home Integrated Care Pathway)

Appendix A

Asthma Protocol (Integrated Care Pathways)

The North West London Hospitals NHS Trust

ADULT ACUTE ASTHMA PROTOCOL

CONSULTANT

PATIENT STICKER

NAMED NURSE

ESSENTIAL INFORMATION FOR ASTHMA ADMISSIONS

- **PEFR actual** ______________ **l/min**
- **PEFR best** ______________ **l/min**

or

- **PEFR predicted** ______________ **l/min**
- **Number of Asthma-related hospital admissions in last year** ______________

Predicted Peak Flow values:

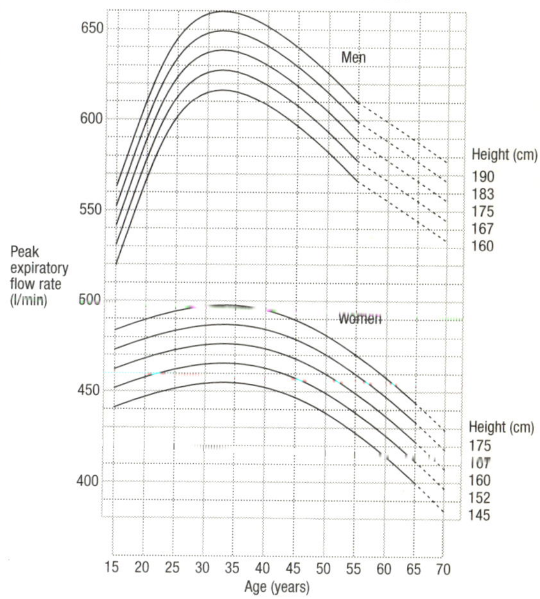

ADDITIONAL DIAGNOSIS/PROBLEMS

Diabetes and high blood pressure may be aggravated by steroid therapy
Other co-morbidities may interfere with management

ANTICIPATED LENGTH OF STAY	**2 NIGHTS**
Date admitted	Date discharged
Time admission	

SUMMARY OF GUIDELINES FOR USE: ALL SECTIONS SHOULD BE ADDRESSED. NONE SHOULD BE LEFT BLANK.

- Enter any extra care provided to show that needs not covered by the protocol have been addressed
- The protocol is *not cast in stone*. If it is appropriate to vary care: state in what way the patient's care will vary; explain the reason for the variance; describe what action is taken as a result
- To meet legal requirements documentation should be accurate and comprehensive

ACUTE ASTHMA – IMMEDIATE MANAGEMENT GUIDELINES

ASSESS FOR IMPORTANT SIGNS AND SYMPTOMS:

The presence of any of the following indicate a severe attack:

- Inability to speak sentences
- Pulse > 110/min
- Respiratory rate > 25/min
- PEFR < 200 L/min or < 50% of predicted

IF PRESENT OR PATIENT DETERIORATES CONSIDER REFERRAL TO ITU:

CYANOSIS
EXHAUSTION
CONFUSION
BRADYCARDIA
SILENT CHEST
PEFR <33% of best or predicted

IMMEDIATE INVESTIGATIONS (All patients)

- PEFR (predicted or best and actual)
- Arterial Blood Gases (ABG)
  The following indicate severe asthma:
  P_aO_2 < 8kPa irrespective of Oxygen treatment
  P_aCO_2, which is normal (5–6kPa) or high
  A low pH < 7.35
- Chest X-ray (NB portable often safest)
- Electrolytes particularly K+

IMMEDIATE MANAGEMENT (Points 1–4 should be performed simultaneously)

1. Oxygen 60% all patients
2. High dose B2 agonists (5 mg Salbutamol or 10 mg terbutaline) delivered by Oxygen nebuliser flow rate 6–8 l/min. These can be repeated as often as necessary and may be continuous.
3. Monitor response (pulse, resp rate, O_2 sats & PEFR)
4. Steroids 40–60 mg oral Prednisolone and 200 mg IV Hydrocortisone within 1 hour of admission.
   Note diabetes and high blood pressure may be aggravated by steroid therapy
5. Antibiotics should only be prescribed if one or more of the following are present: fever, infected sputum, high white cell count and/or X-ray consolidation
   Note: antibiotics are overused in asthma management.

- **If there are life threatening features or poor initial response add 500 mcg Ipratropium to nebulised B_2 agonists. Aminophylline infusion at 0.5 mg/kg/hour and cardiac monitor patients.**

N.B. DO NOT GIVE BOLUS THEOPHYLLINES TO PATIENTS TAKING ORAL THEOPHYLLINES

ACUTE ASTHMA PROTOCOL – Guidance for use

This protocol and the Adult Inpatient Assessment Record form the complete multidisciplinary patient record of care.

- All sections should be addressed. None should be left blank.
- Record on the protocol any extra care provided to show that all needs have been addressed.
- Use the Multidisciplinary Progress Notes to evaluate care and patient's response. Insert extra pages as necessary.
- The protocol is *not cast in stone*. If it is appropriate to vary care: explain the reason; describe what action is taken as a result.
- To meet legal requirements documentation should be accurate and comprehensive.
- Following discharge this protocol will be filed in the medical notes.

Milestones

- These are national standards for asthma care.
- This information is collected for clinical audit purposes to continually improve care.
- Tick the box if the patient meets the milestone or record the reason why the patient did not meet the milestone.

Inhaler Technique Advice

Several types of inhaler device are currently on the market. The two main types used within the trust are metered dose inhalers (MDIs) and Turbohalers. For other devices and advice, check the package insert for administration technique or ask your ward pharmacist or physiotherapist.

	Metered Dose Inhalers	**Turbohalers**
Drugs available	• Salbutamol (Ventolin®) • Beclomethasone 50/100/250 (Becotide®) • Ipratropium (Atrovent®) • Salmeterol (Serevent®)	• Terbutaline (Bricanyl®) • Budesonide 100/200/400 (Pulmicort®) • Eformoterol (Oxis®)
Usual dose	2–4 puffs PRN for Relievers BD–QDS for others	1–2 doses PRN for Relievers BD–QDS for others
Formulation	Drug suspended in a gas, usually CFC-free.	Dry powder inhaler.
Inhaler technique	1. Shake inhaler 2. Remove cap 3. Insert inhaler into mouth, form a seal and breathe through mouth 4. At the beginning of the next breath in press down on canister to release dose and breathe in deeply. 5. Hold breath for up to 10 seconds, if possible.	1. Remove cap 2. Turn dial anti-clockwise and back until 'click' is heard. The dose is now ready. 3. Insert inhaler into mouth, form a seal. 4. Breathe in deeply through mouth to inhale dose. **Note:** Patients using this inhaler will feel no after-taste.
Spacer device	1. Shake inhaler and remove cap 2. Insert inhaler into Volumatic 3. Place Volumatic into mouth and form a seal 4. Press down on canister to release dose 5. Breathe deeply through Volumatic for at least 2 breaths or 10 secs	Not required

Hints and Tips

- Rinse the mouth out with water after taking a steroid preventer inhaler to help prevent oral thrush.
- Volumatics can be rinsed out with water and left to dry naturally. They should be changed every 6–12 months.
- Turbohalers have a window that shows a red line when they need to be replaced. MDIs will simply 'feel light'.

Patient name **DAY 1** Hospital no

MILESTONES/OUTCOMES	MET	If no please give reason and action
• Oral or IV steroids given < 1 hour	❑	
• Inhaled steroids commenced	❑	
• SaO_2 >95% on O_2	❑	
• PEFR recorded at least 4 hourly	❑	

ASSESSMENT		Yes	No
• Unable to speak sentences		❑	❑
• Central cyanosis		❑	❑
• Arterial saturation < 95% on O_2		❑	❑
• Tachycardia > 110/mins		❑	❑
• Respiratory rate > 25/min		❑	❑
• Evidence of CO_2 retention	**If Yes refer to ITU Registrar**	❑	❑
• Poor level of consciousness	**If Yes refer to ITU Registrar**	❑	❑

• Observations: TPR and BP 6 hourly (if stable)
Peak Flow pre and post nebuliser
Pulse Oximetry (O_2 concentration ______ %)

Urinalysis for glucose on admission ______________________________

INVESTIGATIONS	Yes	No	**Comments**		
• Chest X-ray	❑	❑	Pneumothorax	Consolidation	Normal
• Sputum for culture	❑	❑	Hyperexpanded		
• FBC	❑	❑			
• U&Es	❑	❑			
• Repeat ABGs **IF**	❑	❑	Ph	PCO_2	PO_2
Initially abnormal or O_2 sats on air < 92%			HCO_3		
• Theophylline levels if relevant:	❑	❑			

DRUGS	Yes	No
• Commence inhaled steroids	❑	❑

OTHER MANAGEMENT		Yes	No
• **Oxygen therapy** (in high concentrations as necessary consider humidification)	_______ %	❑	❑
• **Refer to physio**		❑	❑
• **Care plan** discussed and explained to patient by:	______________________ (sign)		

ADDITIONAL INFORMATION

RGN: AM PM Night

Patient name Hospital no

Date and Time	**MULTIDISCIPLINARY PROGRESS NOTES**	*Signature and Profession*

Patient name **DAY 2** Hospital no

MILESTONES/OUTCOMES	MET	If no please give reason
• Inhaled steroids commenced	❑	
• PEFR recorded at least 4 hourly	❑	
• Converted to inhalers	❑	

ASSESSMENT	Better	Same	Worse
• Nocturnal breathlessness (ask the patient)	❑	❑	❑
• Able to speak full sentences (ask the patient)	❑	❑	❑
• Wheeze (ask the patient)	❑	❑	❑
• Cough (ask the patient)	❑	❑	❑

• Observations: TPR and BP 6 hourly
Peak Flow pre and post nebuliser
Daily Oxygen Saturations

INVESTIGATIONS	Yes	No	Comments
• Chest X-ray *If not already taken or low on admission*	❑	❑	

DRUGS	Yes	No
• Commence inhaled steroids (with device most suited to patient see page 2)	❑	❑
• Continue with oral steroids	❑	❑
• Commence Inhaled B_2 agonists and discontinue nebulisers **IF all** below met:		
– Peak Flow plateaued	❑	❑
– Morning Dip < 20% of highest PEFR	❑	❑
– O_2 saturation on air > 95%	❑	❑

MANAGEMENT	Yes	No
• **Care plan** discussed and explained to patient by: ______________________ (sign)		
• **Disease Management:** Discuss management of disease, check understanding Asthma leaflets given	❑	❑
• **Inhaler Technique:** Check technique and record: (see guidance on page 3)		
Drug: Device: Competent technique? (if not competent seek advice from physio)	❑	❑
• **Smoking:** If patient smokes discuss ways/help to give up. Advice leaflet given	❑	❑

ADDITIONAL INFORMATION

RGN: AM PM Night

Patient name Hospital no

Date and Time	**MULTIDISCIPLINARY PROGRESS NOTES**	*Signature and Profession*

Patient name **DAY 3** Hospital no

MILESTONES/DISCHARGE OUTCOMES	MET	If no please give reason
• Inhaled steroids commenced	❑	
• Peak Flow plateaued with Morning dips < 20% of highest PEFR following 24 hrs on Inhaled B_2 agonists	❑	
• Stable Peak Flow consistent with previous values	❑	
• Satisfactory inhaler technique	❑	
• Commenced on inhalers 24–48 hrs pre discharge	❑	
• Smokers given cessation advice	❑	
• Oral steroids prescribed for discharge	❑	
• OPA arranged	❑	

• Peak Flow: ______________________ U+E (if on Diuretics/Steroids) ____________________________

ASSESSMENT	Better	Same	Worse
• Nocturnal breathlessness (ask the patient)	❑	❑	❑
• Able to speak full sentences (ask the patient)	❑	❑	❑
• Wheeze (ask the patient)	❑	❑	❑
• Cough (ask the patient)	❑	❑	❑

• Observations: TPR and BP 6 hourly
Peak Flow
Daily Oxygen Saturations

INVESTIGATIONS

DRUGS	Yes	No
• Commence Inhaled B_2 agonists and discontinue nebulisers **IF all** below met:		
– Peak Flow plateaued	❑	❑
– Morning Dip < 20% of highest PEFR	❑	❑
– O_2 saturation on air > 95%	❑	❑
Inhaled B_2 agonists commenced	❑	❑
• TTAs Ordered (include short course of Prednisolone 2/52)	❑	❑

MANAGEMENT	Yes	No
• **Inhaler:** Check technique (see page 3)	❑	❑
• **Discharge:** If patient meets all discharge criteria	❑	❑

ADDITIONAL INFORMATION

RGN: AM PM Night

Patient name

Hospital no

Date and Time	**MULTIDISCIPLINARY PROGRESS NOTES**	*Signature and Profession*

Patient name **DAY 4** Hospital no

MILESTONES/DISCHARGE OUTCOMES MET If no please give reason

- Peak Flow plateaued with Morning dips < 20% of highest PEFR following 24 hrs on Inhaled B_2 agonists ❑
- Stable Peak Flow consistent with previous values ❑
- Satisfactory inhaler technique ❑
- Commenced on inhalers 24–48 hrs pre discharge ❑
- Smokers given cessation advice ❑
- Oral steroids prescribed for discharge ❑
- OPA arranged ❑
- Peak Flow: ______________ U+E (if on Diuretics/Steroids) ______________

ASSESSMENT

	Better	Same	Worse
• Nocturnal breathlessness (ask the patient)	❑	❑	❑
• Able to speak full sentences (ask the patient)	❑	❑	❑
• Wheeze (ask the patient)	❑	❑	❑
• Cough (ask the patient)	❑	❑	❑

- Observations: Peak Flow
  Daily Oxygen Saturations

DRUGS

	Yes	No
• TTAs Ordered (include short course of Prednisolone 2/52)	❑	❑

MANAGEMENT

	Yes	No
• Care plan discussed and explained to patient by: ______________ (sign)	❑	❑
• **Discharge:** Short course of Prednisolone 2/52 (patient involved with plan)	❑	❑
Outpatient appointment made with Chest Clinic	❑	❑

If discharge outcomes are not met and admission continues, record care on continuation sheets

ADDITIONAL INFORMATION

RGN: AM PM Night

Patient name Hospital no

Date and Time	**MULTIDISCIPLINARY PROGRESS NOTES**	*Signature and Profession*

Asthma Protocol Audit Form

This page is to be completed on discharge and returned to the Quality Department

Patient Sticker

Consultant

Discharge ward

Date of Admission ______________________

Day One	Yes	No	If any milestone not met complete reason why not met
• Oral or IV steroids given < 1 hour	❑	❑	Reason:
• Inhaled steroids commenced	❑	❑	
• SaO_2 > 95% on O_2	❑	❑	
• PEFR recorded at least 4 hourly	❑	❑	

Day Two	Yes	No	If any milestone not met complete reason why not met
• Inhaled steroids continued	❑	❑	Reason:
• PEFR recorded at least 4 hourly	❑	❑	
• Converted to inhalers	❑	❑	

Day Three	Yes	No	If any milestone not met complete reason why not met
• Competent inhaler technique	❑	❑	Reason:
• PEFR recorded at least 6 hourly	❑	❑	
• Patient discharged	❑	❑	

Day Four	Yes	No	If any milestone not met complete reason why not met
• Patient discharged	❑	❑	Reason:

Design criteria (complete for **all patients** whenever they were discharged)

	Yes	No
• Peak Flow plateaued	❑	❑
• Morning dips < 20% of highest	❑	❑
• Stable PEFR consistent normal	❑	❑
• Satisfactory inhaler technique	❑	❑
• On inhalers 24–48 hrs pre discharge	❑	❑
• Smokers given cessation advice	❑	❑
• Oral steroids in TTAs	❑	❑
• OPA arranged	❑	❑

Date of discharge ______________________

This page does not form part of the patient's record of care. The information is confidential and will be used to evaluate care, and improve the patients' experience.

Thank you.

Appendix B

Collaborative Care IV Protocol (Hospital at Home Integrated Care Pathways)

Central Middlesex Hospital

ADMINISTRATION OF INTRAVENOUS ANTIBIOTICS COLLABORATIVE CARE TEAM

CRITERIA FOR CCT	Yes	No
• Patient over 18 years old	❑	❑
• No coincidental medical/surgical problems requiring admission	❑	❑
• No adverse social circumstances	❑	❑
• No possible compliance problems with home treatment	❑	❑
• No past medical history of anaphylaxis	❑	❑
• Patient able to transfer independently	❑	❑
• Patient has telephone access	❑	❑
• Cannula or PICC line in situ	❑	❑
• First dose of intravenous antibiotics given with no adverse reaction on hospital site	❑	❑

COMPLETE THE FOLLOWING SECTION IF SUITABLE FOR REFERRAL TO CCT
Contact CCT **Mon–Sun 8am–5pm** on Ext 2233, and fax (2667) through front sheet

Patient Details

Name Hospital No. Episode No.

General Practitioner Telephone

Date of admission and/or discharge Referral Source

Diagnosis

Allergies

Complete Anaphylaxis Risk Assessment Tool overleaf ❑

Current status Mobility

Self care

Pressure areas

Baseline Observations

Temp _____ Pulse ______ B/P _____ Resps _____ BM ______ Pain Score (0–10) _____

Investigations

Wound swab	Result	________________
Bloods		
U & Es	Result	________________
FBC	Result	________________
CRP	Result	________________
ESR	Result	________________
Other	Result	________________

Antibiotic Therapy (Discuss antibiotic regime with Microbiologist Dr Shafi and prescribe on drug chart)

Anticipated length of treatment ____________________

Supply of Equipment/Drugs

Arrange supply of the following: Drugs ❑ Inpatient Drug Chart ❑ Diluents ❑ Saline (flush) ❑ Needles ❑ Syringes ❑ Mediswabs ❑ Gloves ❑ Sharps bin ❑

Other Management/Significant Information

Follow up arrangements

Contact Details To be discharged under the care of

Name ____________________ Team ____________________ Bleep No ____________________

ANAPHYLAXIS RISK ASSESSMENT TOOL

To be completed before the patient is discharged from hospital

	Yes	No
Has the patient received the prescribed drug previously?	❑	❑
Were there any signs of an anaphylactic reaction?	❑	❑
If yes, discuss with Doctor		
Are all the patient's current medications listed?	❑	❑
If no, update the records		
Is the patient allergic to anything?	❑	❑
If yes, document the substance and the symptoms of allergy the patient experienced		
Does the patient have a history of any allergic conditions such as asthma, hayfever, skin reactions eg eczema?	❑	❑
Is there cross sensitivity between the drug to be administered and the medications/food that caused a previous reaction?	❑	❑
Check with pharmacist/Dr if unsure		
Is the patient taking any beta blockers, tricyclic antidepressants or MAOIs?	❑	❑
If yes, patient requires referral for specific anaphylaxis prescription (Half doses of Adrenaline are recommended for patients on these drugs)		
Patient referred to: Doctor ____________________		
Dose prescribed on drug chart	❑	❑
Adrenaline dose to give in emergency ____________________		
Comments on any actions taken		

SIGNATURE	POSITION	DATE

MANAGEMENT OF ANAPHYLAXIS IN THE COMMUNITY

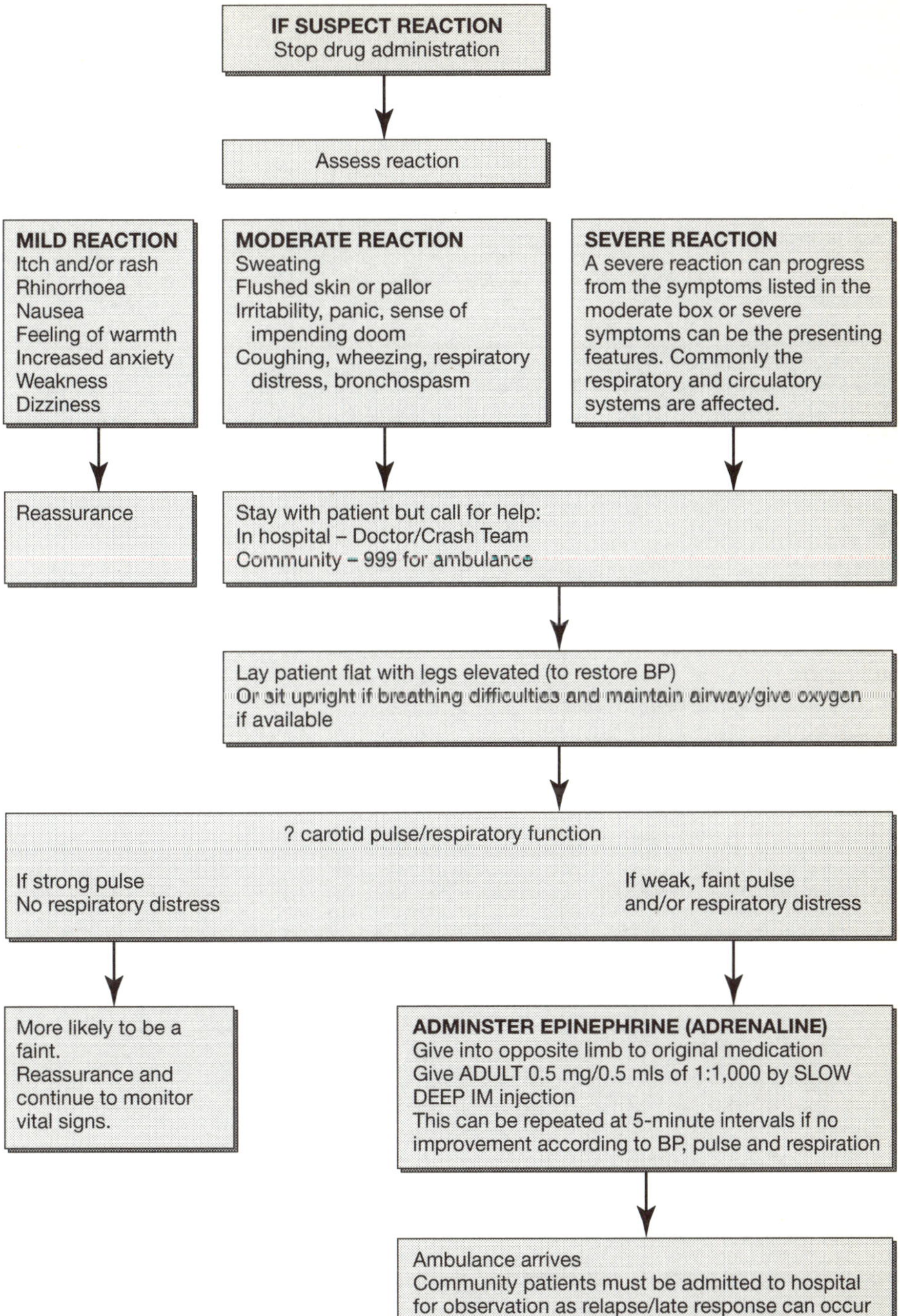

Patient name Hospital No.

TREATMENT PLAN **DAY 1 OF HOME TREATMENT**

MILESTONES/OUTCOMES	MET	If no please give reason
• Patient has a clear understanding of their condition and treatment plan	❑	
• Patient coping with home treatment	❑	
• Medical condition stable	❑	
• Appropriate referrals made (i.e. District Nurses, other)	❑	
• Anaphylaxis kit in patient's home	❑	
• Location of anaphylaxis kit ____________________		

ASSESSMENT	Yes	No
• Temperature ________ Pulse ________ Other _________ Pain score (0–10) ______		
• Site of infection assessed: Improved/No change/Deteriorated		
• IV access assessed for redness, pain, swelling, leakage Action taken:	❑	❑
• Is patient reporting signs of adverse reaction to drugs Action taken:	❑	❑
• Wound care given and chart completed	❑	❑

DRUGS	Yes	No
• Antibiotics Date and time of first dose ____________________________	❑	❑
• Analgesia	❑	❑

MANAGEMENT	Yes	No
• Care plan discussed and explained to patient by: ______________________________ (sign)		
• Patient given contact names and telephone numbers by: ________________________ (sign)		
• Disease Management: Check understanding	❑	❑

SIGNATURE	POSITION	DATE

Patient name | Hospital No.

TREATMENT PLAN | **DAY 2 OF HOME TREATMENT**

MILESTONES/OUTCOMES	MET	If no please give reason
• Patient coping with home treatment	❑	
• Medical condition stable	❑	
• Signs of reduced infection	❑	

ASSESSMENT	Yes	No
• Temperature ________ Pulse ________ Other _________ Pain score (0–10) ______		
• Site of infection assessed:		
No change/deterioration	❑	❑
Rash with blistering	❑	❑
Pain increasing	❑	❑
Persistent pyrexia	❑	❑
Drowsiness	❑	❑
Diarrhoea and vomiting	❑	❑
Blackish discoloration to wound/skin	❑	❑
If yes to any of the above, contact Hospital Team for advice		
• IV access assessed for redness, pain, swelling, leakage Action taken:	❑	❑
• Is patient reporting signs of adverse reaction to drugs Action taken:	❑	❑
• Wound care given and chart completed	❑	❑

DRUGS	Yes	No
• Antibiotics	❑	❑
• Analgesia	❑	❑

SIGNATURE	POSITION	DATE

Patient name

Hospital No.

TREATMENT PLAN

DAY 3 OF HOME TREATMENT

MILESTONES/OUTCOMES	MET	If no please give reason
• Antibiotic therapy reviewed	❑	

ASSESSMENT	Yes	No
• Temperature ________ Pulse ________ Other __________ Pain score (0–10) ______		
• Site of infection assessed: Improved/No change/Deteriorated		
• IV access assessed for redness, pain, swelling, leakage Action taken:	❑	❑
• Is patient reporting signs of adverse reaction to drugs Action taken:	❑	❑
• Wound care given and chart completed	❑	❑

DRUGS	Yes	No
• Antibiotics	❑	❑
• Analgesia	❑	❑

SIGNATURE	POSITION	DATE

Patient name | Hospital No.

TREATMENT PLAN | **DAY 4 OF HOME TREATMENT**

MILESTONES/OUTCOMES	MET	If no please give reason
• Site of infection improving	❑	

ASSESSMENT (Yes / No)

- Temperature ________ Pulse ________ Other __________ Pain score (0–10) ______
- Site of infection assessed: Improved/No change/Deteriorated
- IV access assessed for redness, pain, swelling, leakage — Yes ❑ No ❑
  Action taken:
- Is patient reporting signs of adverse reaction to drugs — Yes ❑ No ❑
  Action taken:
- Wound care given and chart completed — Yes ❑ No ❑

DRUGS	Yes	No
• Antibiotics	❑	❑
• Analgesia	❑	❑

SIGNATURE	POSITION	DATE

Patient name

Hospital No.

TREATMENT PLAN

DAY 5 OF HOME TREATMENT

MILESTONES/OUTCOMES	MET	If no please give reason
• Site of infection improving	❑	

ASSESSMENT	Yes	No
• Temperature ________ Pulse ________ Other __________ Pain score (0–10) ______		
• Site of infection assessed: Improved/No change/Deteriorated		
• IV access assessed for redness, pain, swelling, leakage Action taken:	❑	❑
• Is patient reporting signs of adverse reaction to drugs Action taken:	❑	❑
• Wound care given and chart completed	❑	❑

DRUGS	Yes	No
• Antibiotics	❑	❑
• Analgesia	❑	❑

SIGNATURE	POSITION	DATE

Patient name   Hospital No.

TREATMENT PLAN   **DAY 6 OF HOME TREATMENT**

MILESTONES/OUTCOMES	MET	If no please give reason
• Site of infection improving	❑	

ASSESSMENT

	Yes	No
• Temperature ________ Pulse ________ Other __________ Pain score (0–10) ______		
• Site of infection assessed: Improved/No change/Deteriorated		
• IV access assessed for redness, pain, swelling, leakage Action taken:	❑	❑
• Is patient reporting signs of adverse reaction to drugs Action taken:	❑	❑
• Wound care given and chart completed	❑	❑

DRUGS

	Yes	No
• Antibiotics	❑	❑
• Analgesia	❑	❑

SIGNATURE	POSITION	DATE

Patient name | Hospital No.

TREATMENT PLAN | **DAY 7 OF HOME TREATMENT**

MILESTONES/OUTCOMES	MET	If no please give reason
• Patient discussed with Medical/A & E Team	❑	
• GP informed of outcome and any follow up required	❑	

ASSESSMENT	Yes	No
• Temperature ________ Pulse ________ Other _________ Pain score (0–10) ______		
• Site of infection assessed: Improved/No change/Deteriorated		
• IV access assessed for redness, pain, swelling, leakage Action taken:	❑	❑
• Is patient reporting signs of adverse reaction to drugs Action taken:	❑	❑
• Wound care given and chart completed	❑	❑

DISCHARGE	Yes	No
• Last dose of IVs given	❑	❑
• Patient discussed with Medical/A & E team and discharged to GP	❑	❑
• GP informed of outcome and any follow up required	❑	❑
• Cannula/PICC removed	❑	❑
• Home anaphylaxis kit returned to CCT store	❑	❑
• Sharps bin locked and returned to Central Middlesex Hospital for disposal	❑	❑
• Excess medication disposed of according to policy	❑	❑
• All equipment returned to CCT	❑	❑

SIGNATURE	POSITION	DATE

Patient name

Hospital No.

DRESSING PLAN

Aim: Protection Debridement Deslough Granulation Exudate Management

PRESCRIPTION (Review effectiveness regularly) Give name and size of product	**Initial Dressing Plan**	**Dressing Plan changed Date ____________**
Cleansing solution		
Debridement/Deslough		
Topical application		
Primary contact product		
Secondary contact product		
Fixative (If strike through occurs review dressing)		
Isolated infection		

SIGNATURE	POSITION	DATE

PLEASE INDICATE LOCATION OF WOUND

Patient name

Hospital No.

WOUND ASSESSMENT CHART

Date	Length cm	Width cm	Depth cm	Appearance		Infection	Exudate	Initial
				Wound	Surrounding skin			
Baseline								

Give maximum dimensions for length, depth and width

WOUND APPEARANCE

PINK	Epithelialising	
RED	Granulating	
YELLOW	Sloughy	
BLACK	Necrotic	
Skin	Macerated	Oedematous
	Erythema	Fragile
	Dry/scaly	Healthy/intact

INFECTION

Tick for yes if any of the following present:

- Granulation tissue bleeds easily ❑
- Increased odour/exudate level ❑
- Healing rates slower than anticipated ❑

Wound breakdown
S = Swab taken + sent

EXUDATE

Amount:	High	Medium Low
Type:	Blood	Serous
Odour:	Offensive/None	

HOME INTRAVENOUS DRUG ADMINISTRATION SERVICE
INFORMATION FOR PATIENTS
CANNULAS

It has been decided that you may continue your intravenous (into a vein) treatment at home. In order to enable us to give you your treatment into a vein, it is necessary for you to have a small hollow plastic tube inserted into your hand/arm. This plastic tube is called a CANNULA.

The cannula goes through your skin and into a vein where it stays to allow us to give your medicines directly into your blood stream. You will have a waterproof dressing over the cannula to help keep it in place.

As the cannula is sitting in a vein, there is a risk of bleeding if the cannula becomes accidentally dislodged. THERE IS NO NEED TO PANIC if this does happen. Usually any bleeding will stop within a few minutes with pressure.

IF YOUR CANNULA COMES OUT:

- Apply pressure to the area with cotton wool, gauze or a tissue
- Maintain this pressure until the bleeding has completely stopped
- Once the bleeding has stopped apply a plaster
- If the bleeding has stopped, there is no need to call anyone.

The nurse who visits you for your next treatment will replace the cannula with a new one.

IF THE BLEEDING DOESN'T STOP:

- Keep applying pressure to the area
- Lift your arm above your head
- Telephone the team of nurses looking after you:

During the daytime between 08.00 and 17.00 contact CCT on
020 8453 2233
or
During the evening and night between 17.00 and 08.00,
contact Senior Nurse on call
020 8965 5733 and ask for bleep 345

PLEASE DETACH AND GIVE TO PATIENT